Food Remedies

by Florence Daniel

PREFACE

There is a sentence in the Talmud to the effect that the Kingdom of God is nigh when the teacher gives the name of the author of the information that he is passing on. With every desire to fulfil the rabbinical precept and acknowledge the sources of this booklet, I find myself in a quandary. If I make my acknowledgments duly I must begin with my grandmother and Culpeper's Herbal. Following upon those come the results of my own and friends' practical experience. After this I should, perhaps, give a list of the periodicals from whose pages I have culled much helpful information. But as space and memory preclude individual mention I must content myself with this general acknowledgment. Lastly, I desire to record my thanks to Dr. Fernie, whose Meals Medicinal, a large and exhaustive collection of facts about food, has afforded not the least valuable assistance. F. D.

FOOD REMEDIES

PART I.--INTRODUCTORY

While there is Fruit there is hope.

While there is life--and fruit--there is hope. When this truth is realised by the laity nine hundred and ninety-nine out of every thousand professors of the healing art will be obliged to abandon their profession and take to fruit-growing for a living.

Many people have heard vaguely of the "grape cure" for diseases arising from over-feeding, and the lemon cure for rheumatism, but for the most part these "cures" remain mere names. Nevertheless it is almost incredible to the uninitiated what may be accomplished by the abandonment for a time of every kind of food in favour of fruit. Of course, such a proceeding should not be entered upon in a careless or random fashion. Too sudden changes of habit are apt to be attended with disturbances that discourage the patient, and cause him to lose patience and abandon the treatment without giving it a fair trial. In countries where the "grape cure" is practised the patient starts by taking one pound of grapes each day, which quantity is gradually increased until he can consume six pounds. As the quantity of grapes is increased that of the ordinary food is decreased, until at last the patient lives on nothing but grapes.[1] I have not visited a "grape cure" centre in person, but I have read that it is not only persons suffering from the effects of over-feeding who find salvation in the "grape cure," but that consumptive patients thrive and even put on weight under it.

The Herald of Health stated, some few years back, that in the South of France where the "grape cure" is practised consumptive patients are fed on grapes alone, and become quite strong and well in a year or two. And I have myself known wonderful cures to follow on the adoption of a fruitarian dietary in cases of cancer, tumour, gout, eczema, all kinds of inflammatory complaints, and wounds that refused to heal.

H. Benjafield, M.B., writing in the Herald of Health, says: "Garrod, the great London authority on gout, advises his patients to take oranges, lemons, strawberries, grapes, apples, pears, etc. Tardieu, the great French authority, maintains that the salts of potash found so plentifully in fruits are the chief agents in purifying the blood from these rheumatic and gouty poisons.... Dr. Buzzard advises the scorbutic to take fruit morning, noon, and night. Fresh lemon juice in the form of lemonade is to be his ordinary drink; the existence of diarrhoea should be no reason for withholding it." The writer goes on to show that headache, indigestion, constipation, and all other complaints that result from the sluggish action of bowels and liver can never be cured by the use of artificial fruit salts and drugs.

Salts and acids as found in organised forms are quite different in their effects to the products of the laboratory, notwithstanding that the chemical composition may be shown to be the same. The chemist may be able to manufacture a "fruit juice," but he cannot, as yet, manufacture the actual fruit. The mysterious life force always evades him. Fruit is a vital food, it supplies the body with something over and above the mere elements that the chemist succeeds in isolating by analysis. The vegetable kingdom possesses the power of directly utilising minerals, and it is only in this "live" form that they are fit for the consumption of man. In the consumption of sodium chloride (common table salt), baking powders, and the whole army of mineral drugs and essences, we violate that decree of Nature which ordains that the animal kingdom shall feed upon the vegetable and the vegetable upon the mineral.

FOOTNOTE:

[1] This was the original treatment; now other food is added, although excellent results were obtained under the old regime.

Fruit and the Teeth.

I mention the above because one of the objections that I have heard cited against the free use of fruit is that "the acids act injuriously upon the teeth." Until I became a vegetarian I used to visit a dentist regularly every six months. I had done this for ten years, and nearly every tooth in my gums had its gold filling. The last time I visited the dentist I told him that I had become a vegetarian, and he replied that he rather thought my teeth would decay quicker in future on account of an increased consumption of vegetable acids. But from that day, now nearly six years ago, to the present time, I have never been near a dentist. My teeth seem to have taken a new lease of life. It is a fact that the acids in fruit and vegetables so far from injuring the teeth benefit them. Many of these acids are strongly antiseptic and actually destroy the germs that cause the teeth to decay. On the other hand, they do not attack the enamel of the teeth, while inorganic acids do. Nothing cleanses the teeth so effectually as to thoroughly chew a large and juicy apple.

Fruit is a Food.

Until quite recently the majority of English-speaking people have been accustomed to look upon fruit not as a food, but rather as a sweetmeat, to be eaten merely for pleasure, and therefore very sparingly. It has consequently been banished from its rightful place at the beginning of meals. But fruit is not a "goody," it is a food, and, moreover, a complete food. All vegetable foods (in their natural state) contain all the elements necessary to form a complete food. At a pinch human life might be supported on any one of them. I say "at a pinch" because if the nuts cereals and pulses were ruled out of the dietary it would, for most people, be deficient in fat and proteid (the flesh and muscle-forming element). Nevertheless, fruit alone will sustain life if taken in large quantities with small output of energy on the part of the person living upon it, as witness the "grape cure."[2] The percentage of proteid in grapes is particularly high for fruit.

Those people who desire to make a fruitarian dietary their daily regime cannot do better than take the advice of O. Hashnu Hara, an American writer. He says: "Every adult requires from twelve to sixteen ounces of dry food, free from water, daily. To supply this a quarter of a pound of shelled nuts and three-quarters of a pound of any dried fruit must be used. In addition to this, from two to three pounds of any fresh fruit in season goes to complete the day's allowance. These quantities should be weighed out ... and will sustain a full-grown man in perfect health and vitality. The quantity of ripe fresh fruit may be slightly increased in summer, with a corresponding decrease in the dried fruit."

FOOTNOTE:

[2] Recent years have witnessed a modification of the original cure. Other food is now included, but I have not heard that the results are better.

Objections to Fruit.

Some vegetarians object that it is possible to eat too much fruit, and recommend caution in the use of it to people of nervous temperament, or those who seem predisposed to skin ailments. It is true that the consumption of large quantities of fruit may appear to render the nervous person more irritable, and to increase the external manifestations of a skin disease. But in the latter event the fruit is merely assisting Nature to throw the disease out and off more quickly, while in the former case the real cause lies not in the fruit but in some nerve irritant, tea, for example, the effects of which are more acutely felt under the new regime. The nervous system tends to become much more sensitive upon a vegetarian, especially fruitarian, diet, and people often attribute their increased nervousness and irritability to the diet when it is simply that they now react more quickly to poisons. This is not a bad thing, on the contrary, it shows that the system has become more alert. Under the old regime we tend to store up poisons and impurities in the body, but the effect of a vegetable diet, especially when united with the use of distilled water, is to cause all our diseases and impurities to be expelled outwards and downwards. Tea is a slow poison, and so is coffee except under exceptional conditions when it is used as a medicine, and then it should always be pale-roasted.

Fruit should always be eaten at the beginning of a meal. Again, when the diet consists of a mixture of cooked and uncooked foods, the uncooked should always be eaten first. Also when the meal consists of two courses, a sweet and a savoury dish, sufferers from indigestion should try taking the sweet course first. I have known several cases where this simple expedient has resulted in a complete cessation of the discomfort of which the patient complained.

A Pioneer of Food Remedies.

The pioneer, in England, of the treatment of all sorts and conditions of disease by means of a vegetable (chiefly fruit) dietary was Dr. Lambe, a contemporary of the poet Shelley. His last book appeared in 1815, and in it and the one preceding are recorded some wonderful cures, especially in cases of cancer. It is only fair to add here that in Dr. Lambe's opinion no system of cure is completely efficacious so long as the patient is allowed to drink the ordinary tap or well water. Distilled water was the only drink he advised. But he held it better still not to drink at all if the necessary liquid could be supplied to the body by means of fresh, juicy fruits. He contended that man is not naturally a drinking animal; that his thirst is a morbid symptom, the outcome of a carnivorous diet and other unwholesome habits. And I think that anyone may prove the truth of this for him or herself if he or she will adopt a fruitarian dietary and abstain from the use of salt and other condiments.

I have cited so out-of-date a personage as Dr. Lambe for two reasons. The first is that I know many of the so-called new and unorthodox ideas are more likely to appeal to some readers, if it can be shown that they originated with a duly qualified medical practitioner who recorded the results of his observations and experiments in black and white. The second is that the principles and practices of Dr. Lambe are incorporated with those of the Physical Regeneration Society, a large and ever-increasing body of enthusiasts having its head-quarters in London, to whose annals I must refer those readers who desire up-to-date instances of the efficacy of the use of fruit in disease. Lack of space will not allow me to quote them here.

The Simple Life.

We hear a great deal about the "Simple Life" and "Returning to Nature" nowadays, but most of us are so situated that the proposed simplicity simply spells increased complexity. The "vegetarian chop" costs the housewife more than double the time and labour involved in preparing its fleshly namesake. And when it comes to illness some of the systems of bathing and exercising prescribed by the "naturopath" are infinitely more troublesome to the patient and his friends than the simple expedient of sending for the doctor and taking the prescribed doses. I do not want to be misunderstood here. I am not condemning treatment with water and exercises. On the contrary, I hope to pass on what I have learnt about these methods of treatment. But so many people lack the time, help, and conveniences necessary to carry them out successfully. It is to these that I would say that the patient's cure may be effected just as surely, if more slowly, by means of fruit alone.

Fruit or Fasting.

Treatment of disease by fasting has come into fashion of late, and there is really no lack of proof as to the benefits to be obtained from abstaining entirely from food for a short period. I know of an elderly man who fasts for a fortnight every spring, and gains, not loses, weight during the process! He accounts for this by explaining that certain stored up, undigested food particles come out and are digested while he fasts. Whether this is the correct explanation I do not know, but the fact remains, and it is not by any means a solitary case. Of course, the majority of people lose weight when fasting, but this is very quickly recovered. Now I do not think fasting should be undertaken recklessly, but only under competent direction. But an excellent and safe substitute for a fast is an exclusive fruit diet.

Acute Illness.

The simplest and quickest method of recovering from attacks of acute illness, fevers, inflammatory diseases, etc., is to rest quietly in bed in a warm but well-ventilated room, and to take three meals a day of fresh ripe fruit, grapes by preference. If the grapes are grown out of doors and ripened in the sun so much the better. I have found from two to three pounds of grapes per day sufficient. If there is thirst, barley water flavoured with lemon juice should be taken between the meals.

PART II.--FOODS AND THEIR MEDICINAL USES

Almond.

Almond soup is an excellent substitute for beef-tea for convalescents. It is made by simply blanching and pounding a quarter of a pound of sweet almonds with half a pint of milk, or vegetable stock. Another pint of milk or stock is then to be added and the whole warmed. After this add another pint and a half of stock if the soup is to be a vegetable one, or rice water if milk has been used.

An emulsion of almonds is useful in chest affections. It is made by well macerating the nuts in a nut butter machine, and mixing with orange or lemon juice.

Almonds should always be blanched, that is, skinned by pouring boiling water on the nuts and allowing them to soak for one minute, after which the skins are easily removed. The latter possess irritating properties.

Bitter almonds should not be used as a food. They contain a poison identical with prussic acid.

Apple.

It is hardly possible to take up any newspaper or magazine now a days without happening on advertisements of patent medicines whose chief recommendation is that they "contain phosphorus." They are generally very expensive, but the reader is assured that they are worth ten times the price asked on account of their wonderful properties as nerve and brain foods. The proprietors of these concoctions seemingly flourish like green bay trees and spend many thousands of pounds per annum in advertising. From which it may be deduced that sufferers from nervous exhaustion and brain fag number millions. And surely only a sufferer from brain fag would suffer himself to be led blindly into wasting his money, and still further injuring his health, by buying and swallowing drugs about whose properties and effects he knows absolutely nothing. How much simpler, cheaper, and more enjoyable to eat apples!

The apple contains a larger percentage of phosphorus than any other fruit or vegetable. For this reason it is an invaluable nerve and brain food. Sufferers from nerve and brain exhaustion should eat at least two apples at the beginning of each meal. At the same time they should avoid tea and coffee, and supply their place with barley water or bran tea flavoured with lemon juice, or even apple tea.

Apples are also invaluable to sufferers from the stone or calculus. It has been observed that in cider countries where the natural unsweetened cider is the common beverage, cases of stone are practically unknown. Food-reformers do not deduce from this that the drinking of cider is to be recommended, but that even better results may be obtained from eating the fresh, ripe fruit.

Apples periodically appear upon the tables of carnivorous feeders in the form of apple sauce. This accompanies bilious dishes like roast pork and roast goose. The cook who set this fashion was evidently acquainted with the action of the fruit upon the liver. All sufferers from sluggish livers should eat apples.

Apples will afford much relief to sufferers from gout. The malic acid contained in them neutralises the chalky matter which causes the gouty patient's sufferings.

Apples, when eaten ripe and without the addition of sugar, diminish acidity in the stomach. Certain vegetable salts are converted into alkaline carbonates, and thus correct the acidity.

An old remedy for weak or inflamed eyes is an apple poultice. I am told that in Lancashire they use rotten apples for this purpose, but personally I should prefer them sound.

A good remedy for a sore or relaxed throat is to take a raw ripe apple and scrape it to a fine pulp with a silver teaspoon. Eat this pulp by the spoonful, very slowly, holding it against the back of the throat as long as possible before swallowing.

A diet consisting chiefly of apples has been found an excellent cure for inebriety. Health and strength may be fully maintained upon fine wholemeal unleavened bread, pure dairy or nut butter, and apples.

Apple water or apple tea is an excellent drink for fever patients.

Apples possess tonic properties and provoke appetite for food. Hence the old-fashioned custom of eating an apple before dinner.

Apple Tea.

The following are two good recipes for apple tea:-- (1) Take 2 sound apples, wash, but do not peel, and cut into thin slices. Add some strips of lemon rind. Pour on 1 pint of boiling water (distilled). Strain when cold. (2) Bake 2 apples. Pour over them 1 pint boiling water. Strain when cold.

Asparagus.

Asparagus is said to strengthen and develop the artistic faculties. It also calms palpitation of the heart. It is very helpful to rheumatic patients on account of its salts of potash. It should be steamed, not boiled, otherwise part of the valuable salts are lost.

Banana.

The banana is invaluable in inflammation of all kinds. For this reason it is very useful in cases of typhoid fever, gastritis, peritonitis, etc., and may constitute the only food allowed for a time.

Not only does it actually subdue the inflammation of the intestines, but, in the opinion of at least one authority, as it consists of 95 per cent. nutriment, it does not possess sufficient waste matter to irritate the inflamed spots.

But great care should be taken in its administration. The banana should be thoroughly sound and ripe, and all the stringy portion carefully removed. It should then be mashed and beaten to a cream. In severe cases I think it is better to give this neat, but if not liked by the patient a little lemon juice, well mixed in, may render it more acceptable. It may also be taken with fresh cream.

A friend who has had a very wide experience in illness told me that she was once hurriedly sent for at night to a girl suffering from peritonitis. Not knowing what she might, or might not, find in the way of remedies when she arrived at her destination, my friend took with her some strong barley water, bananas, and an enema syringe. She found the girl lying across the bed screaming, obviously in agony. First of all my friend administered a warm water enema. A pint of plain warm water was injected first, and after this had come away as much warm water as could be got in was injected and then allowed to come away. The object of this was to thoroughly wash out the bowels. Then the barley water was warmed, the bananas mashed, beaten to cream, and mixed in with the barley water. A soothing nutrient lotion was thus prepared, and as much as the patient could bear comfortably was injected in the bowel and retained as long as possible. The effect was magical. The pain subsided, and the patient ultimately recovered.

In the absence of perfectly ripe bananas, baked bananas may be used. But, although better than no fruit at all, cooked fruit is never so valuable as the fresh fruit, if only the latter be perfectly ripe. Bananas should be baked in their skins, and the stringy pieces carefully removed before eating. From twenty minutes to half an hour's slow cooking is required.

Bananas are excellent food for anemic persons on account of the iron they contain. A very palatable way of taking them is with fresh orange juice.

A comparatively old-fashioned remedy, for sprained or bruised places that show a tendency to become inflamed is to apply a plaster of banana skin.

Barley.

Barley is excellent food for the anemic and nervous on account of its richness in iron and phosphoric acid. It is also useful in fevers and all inflammatory diseases, on account of its soothing properties. From the earliest times barley water has been the recognised drink of the sick.

Barley Water.

When using pearl barley for making barley water it must be well washed. The fine white dust that adheres to it is most unwholesome. For this reason the cook is generally directed to first boil the barley for five minutes, and throw this water away. But in this way some of the valuable properties are thrown away with the dirt. The best results are obtained by well washing it in cold water, but this must be done over and over again. Half-a-dozen waters will not be too many. After the last washing the water should be perfectly clear.

When barley water is being used for curative purposes it should be strong. The following recipe is an excellent one. A ?pint of barley to 2?pints water (distilled if possible). Boil for three hours, or until reduced to 2 pints. Strain and add 4 teaspoonfuls fresh lemon juice. Sweeten to taste with pure cane sugar.

Fine Scotch barley is to be preferred to the pearl barley if it can be obtained.

Blackberry.

Fresh blackberries are one of the most effectual cures for diarrhoea known. Mr. Broadbent records the case of a child who was cured by eating an abundance of blackberries after five doctors had tried all the known remedies in vain.

Blackberry Tea.

In the absence of the fresh fruit a tea made of blackberry jelly and hot water (a large tablespoonful of jelly to half a pint water) will be found very useful. A teacupful should be taken at short intervals.

Blackberry Jelly.

To make blackberry jelly get the first fruit of the season if possible, and see that it is ripe or it will yield very little juice. Put it into the preserving pan, crush it, and allow it to simmer slowly until the juice is well drawn out. This will take from three-quarters to one hour. Strain through a jelly bag, or fine clean muslin doubled will do. Then measure the juice, and to every pint allow ?lb. best cane sugar. Return to the pan and boil briskly for from twenty minutes to half an hour. Stir with a wooden spoon and keep well skimmed. To test, put a little of the jelly on a cold plate, and if it sets when cold it is done. While still at boiling point pour into clean, dry, and hot jars, and tie down with parchment covers immediately.

Black Currant.

Black currant tea is one of the oldest of old-fashioned remedies for sore throats and colds. It is made by pouring half a pint of boiling water on to a large tablespoonful of the jelly or jam. To make the jelly use the same recipe as for blackberry jelly.

The fresh juice pressed from the fruit is, of course, better than tea made from the jelly, but as winter is the season of coughs and colds the fruit is least obtainable when most needed.

Brazil Nut.

Brazil nuts are excellent for constipation. They are also a good substitute for suet in puddings. Use 5 oz. nuts to 1 lb. flour. They should be grated in a nut mill or finely chopped.

Beans, Peas, and Lentils.

Beans, peas, and lentils are tabooed by the followers of Dr. Haig, the gout specialist, on account of the belief that they tend to increase the secretion of uric acid. But this evil propensity is stoutly denied by other food-reformers. For myself I am inclined to believe that their supposed indigestibility, etc., arises from the fact that they are generally cooked in hard water. They should be cooked in distilled or boiled and filtered rain water. The addition of lemon juice while cooking renders them much more digestible.

According to Sir Henry Thomson haricot beans are more easily digested than meat by most stomachs. "Consuming weight for weight, the eater feels lighter and less oppressed, as a rule, after the leguminous dish; while the comparative cost is greatly in favour of the latter."

Lentils are the most easily digested of all the pulse foods, and therefore the most suitable for weakly persons. A soup made of distilled water and red lentils may be taken twice a week with advantage. Lentils contain a good percentage of iron, and also phosphates.

Beet.

The red beet is useful in some diseases of the womb, while the white beet is good for the liver. It is laxative and diuretic. The juice mixed with olive oil is also recommended to be applied externally for burns and all kinds of running sores.

Cabbage.

All the varieties of the colewort tribe, including cabbage, cauliflower, brussels-sprouts, broccoli, and curly greens, have been celebrated from very ancient times for their curative virtues in pulmonary complaints. And Athenian doctors prescribed cabbage for nursing mothers. On account of the sulphur contained in them cabbages are good for rheumatic patients. They may be eaten steamed, or, better still, boiled in soft water and the broth only taken. The ordinary boiled cabbage is an indigestible "windy" vegetable, and should never be eaten.

Caraway Seed.

Caraway seeds sharpen the vision, promote the secretion of milk, and are good against hysterical affections. They are also useful in cases of colic. When used to flavour cakes the seeds should be pounded in a mortar, especially if children are to partake thereof.

When used medicinally 20 grains of the powdered seeds may be taken in a wineglassful of hot water. But for children half an ounce of the bruised seeds are to be infused in cold water for six hours, and from 1 to 3 teaspoonfuls of this water given.

A poultice of crushed caraway seeds moistened with hot water is good for sprains.

Caraway seeds are narcotic, and should therefore be used with caution.

Carrot.

Carrots are strongly antiseptic. They are said to be mentally invigorating and nerve restoring. They have the reputation of being very indigestible on account of the fact that they are generally boiled, not steamed. When used medicinally it is best to take the fresh, raw juice. This is easily obtained by grating the carrot finely on a common penny bread grater, and straining and pressing the pulp thus obtained.

Raw carrot juice, or a raw carrot eaten fasting, will expel worms. The cooked carrot is useless for this purpose.

A poultice of fresh carrot pulp will heal ulcers.

Fresh carrot juice is also good for consumptives on account of the large amount of sugar it contains.

Carrots are very good for gouty subjects and for derangements of the liver.

Celery.

Celery is almost a specific for rheumatism, gout, and nervous indigestion. The most useful plants for this purpose are small, not too rapidly grown nor very highly manured.

It may be eaten raw, or steamed, or in soup. Strong celery broth flavoured with parsley is excellent.

Cresses.

All the cresses are anti-scorbutic, that is, useful against the scurvy. The ancient Greeks also believed them to be good for the brain.

The ordinary "mustard and cress" of our salads is good for rheumatic patients, while the water-cress is valuable in cases of tubercular disease. Anemic patients may also eat freely of it on account of the iron it contains. Care should be taken, however, from whence it is procured, as a disease peculiar to sheep but communicable to man may be carried by it. It should not be gathered from streams running through meadows inhabited by sheep.

Chestnut.

Chestnuts, when cooked, are valuable food for persons with weak digestive powers. They should be put on the fire in a saucepan of cold water and cooked for twenty minutes from the time the water first boils. John Evelyn, F.R.S., a seventeenth century writer, says of them: "They are a lusty and masculine food for rustics at all times, and of better nourishment for husbandmen than cole and rusty bacon, yea, or beans to boot."

Cinnamon.

Cinnamon is a very old-fashioned remedy for soothing the pain of internal or unbroken cancer. One prescription is the following: Take 1 lb. of Ceylon sticks. Simmer in a closed vessel with 1 quart of water until the liquid is reduced to 1 pint. Pour off without straining, and shake or stir well before taking. Take half a pint every twenty-four hours. Divide into small doses and take regularly.

Cinnamon has a powerful influence over disease germs, but care must be taken to obtain it pure. It is often adulterated with cassia.

Cinnamon tea may be taken with advantage in cases of consumption, influenza, and pneumonia.

Cocoanut.

Cocoanut is an old and very efficacious remedy for intestinal worms of all kinds. A tablespoonful of freshly-ground cocoanut should be taken at breakfast until the cure is complete. The dessicated cocoanut is useless for curative purposes.

Coffee.

Coffee is a most powerful antiseptic, and therefore very useful as a disinfectant. It has been used as a specific against cholera with marvellous results, and is useful in all cases of intestinal derangement. But only the pale-roasted varieties should be taken, as the roasting develops the poisonous, irritating properties. There is always danger in the roasting of grains or berries on account of the new substances that may be developed.

I do not recommend coffee as a beverage, but as a medicine.

Date.

The nourishing properties of dates are well known. They are easily digested, and for this reason are often recommended to consumptive patients.

According to Dr. Fernie half a pound of dates and half a pint of new milk will make a satisfying repast for a person engaged in sedentary work.

Elderberry.

The elderberry has fallen into neglect of late years, owing to the lazy and disastrous modern habit of substituting the mineral drugs of the chemist for the home-made vegetable remedies of our grandmothers. Nevertheless, the elderberry is one of the most ancient and tried of medicines, held in such great esteem in Germany that, according to the German folk-lore, men should take off their hats in the presence of an elder-tree. In Denmark there is a legend to the effect that the trees are under the protection of a being known as the Elder-Mother, who has been immortalised in one of the fairy tales of Hans Andersen.

The berries of the elder-tree are not palatable enough to be used as a common article of food, but in the days when nearly every garden boasted its elder-tree few housewives omitted to make elderberry wine in due season.

It is not permitted to "food-reformers" to make "wine," but those readers who are fortunate enough to possess an elder-tree might well preserve the juice of the berries against winter coughs and colds.

Preserved Fruit Juice.

The following is E. and B. May's recipe for preserving fruit juice. Put the fruit into a preserving-pan, crush it and allow it to simmer slowly until the juice is well drawn out. This will take about an hour. Press out the juice and strain through a jelly-bag until quite clear. Put the juice back into the pan, and to every quart add a quarter of a pound of best cane sugar. Stir until dissolved. Put the juice into clean, dry bottles. Stand the bottles in a pan of hot water, and when the latter has come to the boil allow the bottles to remain in the boiling water for fifteen minutes. The idea is to bring the juice inside the bottles to boiling point just before sealing up, but not to boil it. See that the bottles are full. Cork immediately on taking out of the pan, and then seal up. To seal mix a little plaster of Paris with water and spread it well over the cork. Let it come a little below the cork so as to exclude all air.

The juice of the elderberry is famous for promoting perspiration, hence its efficacy in the cure of colds. Two tablespoonfuls should be taken at bed-time in a tumbler of hot water.

The juice of the elderberry is excellent in fevers, and is also said to promote longevity.

Elderberry Poultice.

"The leaves of the elder, boiled until they are soft, with a little linseed oil added thereto," laid upon a scarlet cloth and applied, as hot as it can be borne, to piles, has been said to be an infallible remedy. Each time this poultice gets cold it must be renewed for "the space of an hour." At the end of this time the final dressing is to be "bound on," and the patient "put warm to bed." If necessary the whole operation is to be repeated; but the writer assures us that "this hath not yet failed at the first dressing to cure the disease." If any reader desires to try the experiment I would suggest that the leaves be steamed rather than boiled, and pure olive oil used in the place of linseed oil. It must also be remembered that no outward application can be expected to effect a permanent cure, since the presence of piles indicates an effort of Nature to clear out some poison from the system. But if this expulsion is assisted by appropriate means the pain may well be alleviated by external applications. (Pepper should be avoided by sufferers from piles.)

Fig.

A "lump of figs" laid on the boil of King Hezekiah, as recorded in 2 Kings xx. 7, brought about that monarch's recovery. The figs used were doubtless ripe figs, not the dried figs of our grocers.

"This fruit," says Dr. Fernie, "is soft, easily digested, and corrective of strumous disease." The large blue fig may be grown in England, in the milder parts and under a warm wall. The fresh figs were rarely seen at one time outside of the large "high-class" fruit shops, but for the last year or two I have seen them peddled in the streets of London like apples and oranges in due season.

Green figs (not unripe) were commonly eaten by Roman gladiators, which is surely a sufficient tribute to the fruit's strength-giving qualities.

The best way of preparing dried figs for eating is to wash them very quickly in warm water, and steam for twenty minutes or until tender.

Grape.

The special value of the grape lies in the fact that it is a very quick repairer of bodily waste, the grape sugar being taken immediately into the circulation without previous digestion. For this reason is grape juice the best possible food for fever patients, consumptives, and all who are in a weak and debilitated condition. The grapes should be well chewed, the juice and pulp swallowed, and the skin and stones rejected.

In countries where the grape cure is practised, consumptive patients are fed on the sweeter varieties of grape, while those troubled with liver complaints, acid gout, or other effects of over-feeding, take the less sweet kinds.

Dr. Fernie deprecates the use of grapes for the ordinary gouty or rheumatic patient, but with all due deference to that learned authority, I do not believe the fruit exists that is not beneficial to the gouty person. One of the most gouty and rheumatic people I know, a vegetarian who certainly never over-feeds himself, derives great benefit from a few days' almost exclusive diet of grapes.

Cream of tartar, a potash salt obtained from the crust formed upon bottles and casks by grape juice when it is undergoing fermentation in the process of becoming wine, is often used as a medicine. It has been cited as an infallible specific in cases of smallpox, but I do not recommend its use, as it probably gets contaminated with other substances during the process of manufacture. In any case its value cannot be compared with the fresh, ripe fruit. I have little doubt but that an exclusive diet of grapes, combined with warmth, proper bathing, and the absence of drugs, would suffice to cure the most malignant case of smallpox.

Sufferers from malaria may use grapes with great benefit. For this purpose the grapes, with the skins and stones, should be well pounded in a mortar and allowed to stand for three hours. The juice should then be strained off and taken. Or persons with good teeth may eat the grapes, including the skins and stones, if they thoroughly macerate the latter.

In the absence of fresh grapes raisin-tea is a restoring and nourishing drink. Dr. Fernie notes that it is of the same proteid value as milk, if made in the proportions given below. It is much more easily digested than milk, and therefore of great use in gastric complaints. Sufferers from chronic gastritis could not do better than make raisin-tea their sole drink, and bananas their only food for a time.

Raisin Tea.

To make raisin-tea, take half a pound of good raisins and wash well, but quickly, in lukewarm water. Cut up roughly and put into the old-fashioned beef-tea jar with a quart of distilled or boiled and filtered rain water. Cook for four hours, or until the liquid is reduced to 1 pint. Scald a fine hair sieve and press through it all except the skins and stones. If desired a little lemon juice may be added.

Gooseberry.

The juice of green gooseberries "cureth all inflammations," while the red gooseberry is good for bilious subjects. But it has been said that gooseberries are not good for melancholy persons.

Gooseberries are an excellent "spring medicine."

Lavender.

It is very much to be regretted that the nerve-soothing vegetable perfumes of our grandmothers have been superseded, for the most part, by the cheap mineral products of the laboratory. Scents really prepared from the flowers that give them their names are expensive to make, and consequently high-priced. The cheap scents are all mineral concoctions, and their use is more or less injurious. A penny-worth of dried lavender flowers in a muslin bag is even cheaper to buy, inoffensive to smell--which is more than can be said of cheap manufactured scents--and possesses medicinal properties.

Lavender flowers were formerly used for their curative virtues in all disorders of the head and nerves.

An oil, prepared by infusing the crushed lavender flowers in olive oil, is recommended for anointing palsied limbs, and at one time a spirit was prepared from lavender flowers which was known as "palsy drops."

A tea made with hot water and lavender tops will relieve the headache that comes from fatigue.

Dr. Fernie advises 1 dessertspoonful per day of pure lavender water for eczema.

The scent of lavender will keep away flies, fleas, and moths.

Lemon.

Lemons are invaluable in cases of gout, malaria, rheumatism, and scurvy. They are also useful in fevers and liver complaints.

I have found the juice of one lemon taken in a little hot water remove dizzy feelings in the head, accompanied by specks and lights dancing before the eyes, consequent upon the liver being out of order, in half an hour.

The juice of a lemon in hot water may be taken night and morning with advantage by sufferers from rheumatism. In the "lemon cure" for gout and rheumatism, the patients begin with one lemon per day and increase the quantity until they arrive at a dozen or more. But I think this is carrying it to excess. Dr. Fernie recommends the juice of one lemon mixed with an equal proportion of hot water, to be taken pretty frequently, in cases of rheumatic fever.

A prescription for malaria, given in the Lancet, is the following: "Take a full-sized lemon, cut it in thin transverse slices, rind and all, boil these down in an earthenware jar containing a pint and a half of water, until the decoction is reduced to half a pint. Let this cool on the window-sill overnight, and drink it off in the morning."

A Florentine doctor discovered that fresh lemon juice will alleviate the pain of cancerous ulceration of the tongue. His patient sucked slices of lemon.

A German doctor found that fresh lemon juice kills the diptheria bacillus, and advises a gargle of diluted lemon juice to diptheric patients. Such a gargle is excellent for sore throat.

Dr. Fernie recommends lemon juice for nervous palpitation of the heart.

Lemon juice rubbed on to corns will eventually do away with them, and if applied to unbroken chilblains will effect a cure.

Lemon juice is also an old remedy for the removal of freckles and blackheads from the face. It should be rubbed in at bedtime, after washing with warm water.

Lettuce.

Lettuce is noted for its sedative properties, although these are not great in the large, highly-manured, commercial specimens. It is very easily digested, and may, therefore, be eaten by those with whom salads disagree in the ordinary way.

Nettle.

The tender tops of young nettles picked in the spring make a delicious vegetable, somewhat resembling spinach. They are excellent for sufferers from gout and skin eruptions.

Fresh nettle juice is prescribed in doses of from 1 to 2 tablespoonfuls for loss of blood from the lungs, nose, or internal organs.

Nuts.

Nuts are the true substitute for flesh meat. They contain everything in the way of nourishment that meat contains, minus the poisonous constituents of the latter. They are very rich in proteid (flesh and muscle former) and fat. In addition they possess all the constituents that go to make up a perfect food.

Nuts and water form a complete dietary, although I do not suggest that any reader should try it. If he did so he would probably eat too many nuts, not realising how great an amount of nourishment is contained in a concentrated form. No one should eat more than a quarter of a pound of nuts per day, in addition to other food. A pound per day would be more than sufficient if no other food were taken. I have little doubt but that the diet of the future will consist solely of nuts and fresh fruit. After all it is the food most favoured by monkeys, and our teeth and digestive apparatus more nearly resemble those of the monkey than the carnivorous and herbivorous animals so many of us seemingly prefer to imitate.

The chief objection to nuts is supposed to be on account of their indigestibility. But this has its foundation, not in the nut, but in the manner of eating it. I recommend all those people who find nuts indigestible to pay a visit to the Zoo and see how the monkey eats his nuts. He chews and chews and chews. And after that he chews!

I know, alas! that the majority of people do not possess teeth like the monkey, and to these I can only suggest that they macerate their nuts in a nut butter machine. There are several of these machines on the market, and they are stocked by all large "Food-Reform" provision dealers. They cost anything from six or seven shillings. The daily allowance of nuts may be thoroughly macerated and eaten with fruit in the place of cream. Ordinary people may use a nut-mill, which flakes, not macerates, the nuts. But people with bad teeth and a weak digestion will do better to invest in a nut butter machine. I may add that the nuts will not macerate properly unless they are crisp, and to this end they must be put in a warm oven for a short time, just before grinding. I have found new, English-grown walnuts crisp enough without this preparation. But if the nuts are not crisp enough they will simply clog the machine.

Now to our nuts! Almonds are the most nourishing. Next in order come walnuts, hazel or cob nuts, and Brazil nuts. The proteid value of these three does not differ much. After these come the chestnut and cocoanut, and lastly we have the pine kernel. Speaking very roughly, we may liken walnuts, hazel nuts, and Brazil nuts to beef for flesh and muscle-forming value, while pine kernels correspond more nearly to fish. Almonds are nearly double the value of beef.

Nut Cream.

Doctor Fernie recommends the following nut-cream for brain-workers. Pound in a mortar, or mince finely, 3 blanched almonds, 2 walnuts, 2 ounces of pine kernels. Steep overnight in orange or lemon juice.

It should be made fresh daily, and may be used in place of butter.

Oat.

The oat is generally cited as the most nourishing of all the cereals, and a good nerve food. The fine oatmeal gruel of our grandmothers has gone almost entirely out of fashion, but its use might be revived with advantage. Like wheat, it is a complete food. A good preparation of groats (ground oats from which the husk has been entirely removed) may be taken by those who find other preparations indigestible.

Some persons seem unable to take oatmeal, its use being followed by a skin eruption. This is supposed to be due to a special constituent called "avenin," the existence of which, however, is denied by some authorities.

There is little doubt but that persons of weak digestive powers and sedentary habits cannot digest porridge comfortably. In any case quickly-cooked porridge is an abomination.

Olive.

The chief use of the olive, at least in this country, consists in the oil expressed from it. Unfortunately our so-called olive oil is generally cotton-seed oil. Captain Diamond of San Francisco, aged 111, and the oldest living athlete in the world, attributes much of his health to the use of olive oil. But he lays great stress upon the importance of obtaining it pure. Cotton-seed oil consists partly of an indigestible gum, and its continued ingestion tends to produce kidney trouble and heart failure.

A simple test for purity is to use, the suspected sample for oiling floors or furniture. If pure, it will leave a beautiful polish minus grease. But if it contains cotton-seed oil, part of it will evaporate, leaving the gummy portion behind.

When pure olive oil is shaken in a half-filled bottle, the bubbles formed thereby rapidly disappear, but if the sample is adulterated the bubbles continue some time before they burst.

Pure olive oil is pale and a greenish yellow.

If equal volumes of strong nitric acid (this may be obtained from any chemist) and olive oil are mixed together and shaken in a flask the resulting product has a greenish or orange tinge which remains unchanged after standing for ten minutes. But if cotton-seed oil is present, the mixture is reddish in colour, and becomes brown or black on standing.

Olive oil is slightly laxative, and therefore useful to sufferers from constipation. It is also an excellent vermifuge.

Olive oil has been used with great success in the treatment of gall stones. A Dr. Rosenberg reported that of twenty-one cases treated by "the ingestion of a considerable quantity of olive oil, only two failed of complete recovery."

Onion.

The uses of the onion are many and varied. Fresh onion juice promotes perspiration, relieves constipation and bronchitis, induces sleep, is good for cases of scurvy and sufferers from lead colic. It is also excellent for bee and wasp stings.

Onions are noted for their nerve-soothing properties. They are also beautifiers of the complexion. But moderation must be observed in their use or they are apt to disagree. Not everyone can digest onions, although I believe them to be more easily digested raw than cooked.

A raw onion may be rubbed on unbroken chilblains with good results. If broken, the onion should be roasted. The heart of a roasted onion placed in the ear is an old-fashioned remedy for earache.

Raw onions are a powerful antiseptic. They also attract disease germs to themselves, and for this reason may be placed in a sickroom with advantage. Needless to say, they should afterwards be burnt or buried. Culpeper, the ancient herbalist, says that they "draw corruption unto them." It is possibly for this reason that the Vedanta forbids them to devout Hindoos.

Garlic possesses the same properties as the onion, but in a very much stronger degree. Leeks are very much milder than the onion.

Onion Juice.

The following prescription is excellent for sufferers from bronchitis or coughs: Slice a Spanish onion; lay the slices in a basin and sprinkle well with pure cane sugar. Cover the basin tightly and leave for twelve hours. After this time the basin should contain a quantity of juice. Give a teaspoonful every now and then until relief is afforded. If too much be taken it may induce headache and vomiting.

Onion Poultice.

An excellent poultice for the chest may be made by placing one or two English onions in a muslin bag and pounding them to a pulp. This should be renewed every three or four hours, and the chest washed. I have been told that, at the age of six weeks old, I was saved from dying of bronchitis by such an onion poultice applied to the soles of my feet.

Orange.

The orange possesses most of the virtues of the lemon, but in a modified form. But it has the advantage of being more palatable.

The juice of oranges has been observed to exert such a beneficial influence on the blood as to prevent and cure influenza. Taken freely while the attack is on they seemingly prevent the pneumonia that so often follows. By far the quickest way to overcome influenza is to subsist solely on oranges for three or four days. Hot distilled water may be taken in addition.

The peel of the bitter Seville orange is an excellent tonic and remedy in cases of malaria and ague. A drink may be prepared from it according to the prescription under the heading "Lemon."

The "orange cure" is used with great success for consumptive patients, for chest affections of all kinds, for asthma, and some stomach complaints. Oranges are taken freely at every meal. The "navel" kind are generally used.

Herbalists sell dried orange pips to be crushed to a powder and taken in the proportion of 1 teaspoonful to a cup of hot water. This is a harmless sedative, and useful in hysterical affections.

Marmalade Tonic.

A drink made with half a pint of hot water poured over a tablespoonful of good, home-made marmalade will often give relief in cases of neuralgia and pains in the head.

Parsley.

Parsley is useful in cases of menstrual obstruction and diseases of the kidneys. The bruised leaves applied to the breasts of nursing mothers are said to cure painful lumps and threatened abscess. It may also be taken with advantage by cancerous patients. In all these cases parsley may be taken in the form of a soup, in common use among members of the Physical Regeneration Society, which consists of onions, tomatoes, celery, and parsley, stewed together in distilled water.

Dr. Fernie remarks that when uncooked parsley has been eaten to excess it has been observed to produce epilepsy in certain bodily systems. The oil of parsley has also been found useful in cases of epilepsy. This would naturally follow on the homeopathic principle of similars.

Pear.

The pear possesses most of the virtues of the apple. But, unlike the latter, it is credited with producing a constipating effect if eaten without its skin. In an old recipe book I found the following tribute to Bergamot pears. The writer says: "I had for some years been afflicted with the usual symptoms of the stone in the bladder, when meeting with Dr. Lobb's "Treatise of Dissolvents for the Stone and Gravel," I was induced on his recommendation to try Bergamot pears, a dozen or more every day with the rind, when in less than a week I observed a large red flake in my urine, which, on a slight touch, crumbled into the finest powder, and this was the same for several succeeding days. It is ten years since I made the experiment, and I have been quite free from any complaints of that nature ever since. The pears were of the small sort and full of knots."

Pea Nut.

The pea nut--or monkey nut--is especially recommended as a cure for indigestion. I have not been able to find out why. As a matter of fact it is such a highly-concentrated food that, unless taken in very small quantities, it is liable to upset weak digestions. I suspect the secret to lie in the chewing. Almost any kind of nut will cure the habitual indigestion induced by "bolting" the food, if only it be chewed until it is liquid. Hard biscuits will do instead of nuts, although an uncooked food like the nut is the better. But whatever is taken must be "Fletcherised," that is, chewed and chewed and chewed until it is all reduced to liquid.

Pea nuts contain a good deal of oil, and for this reason are recommended for consumptives. They are the cheapest nuts to buy, for the reason that they are not really nuts but beans.

Pine-apple.

Pine-apple juice is the specific for diphtheria. This seems to have been first brought to the notice of Europeans by the fact that negroes living round about the swamps of Louisiana were observed to use it with great success. A writer who records this says: "The patient should be forced to swallow the juice. This fluid is of so pungent and corrosive a nature that it cuts out the diphtheria mucous and causes it to disappear."

The above direction looks satisfactory enough on paper, and it is eminently cheering to read of how the pine-apple juice causes the diphtheria mucous to disappear, but anyone who knows anything about diphtheria knows that to "force" a diphtheria patient to swallow is more easily written about than accomplished. Fortunately I have been able to obtain the following explicit directions from an experienced nurse and mother:

The pine-apple should be cut up and well pounded in a mortar. The juice must then be pressed out and strained through well-scalded muslin. The patient's mouth must be washed out with warm water. The juice may now be given with a silver teaspoon. It is possible that the patient may be quite unable to swallow any of it. If this be so, the juice will serve as a mouth and throat wash. It will gradually dissolve the membrane, and enable it to be scraped gently away with the spoon. The juice should be given, and the throat scraped as far down as the nurse can reach, as often as the patient can bear it. The time will come, sooner or later, when the juice is swallowed. No other food should be given. The nurse may have to work away for some hours before any juice is swallowed, but my friend assures me that if the scraping be done gently and skilfully, even children will bear it patiently. Only a silver or bone spoon should be used, and, needless to say, it must be well scalded in boiling water in the intervals of using.

It is a remarkable fact that while pine-apple juice exercises this remarkable corrosive power upon diseased mucous, its effect upon the most delicate, healthy membrane is absolutely harmless. I have seen sweet pine-apple juice given to six-months-old babies as a supplement to the mother's milk, with excellent results.

Dr. Hillier, writing in the Herald of Health in 1897, says "Sliced pine-apples, laid in pure honey for a day or two, when used in moderation, will relieve the human being from chronic impaction of the bowels, reestablish peristaltic motion, and induce perfect digestion."

"A slice of fresh pine-apple," writes Dr. Fernie, "is about as wise a thing as one can take by way of dessert after a substantial meal." This is because fresh pine-apple juice has been found to act upon animal food in very much the same way that the gastric juice acts within the stomach. But vegetarians should eat fresh fruit at the beginning of meals rather than at the end.

The pine-apple is useful in all ordinary cases of sore-throat.

One pine-apple of average size should yield half a pint of juice.

Tinned or cooked pine-apple is useless for curative purposes.

Pine Kernel.

Pine kernels are recommended to those who find other nuts difficult to digest. They are the most easily digested of all the nuts. They are often used for cooking in the place of suet, being very oily.

Plum, Prune.

The disfavour with which "stone fruits," especially plums, are generally regarded owes its being to the fact that they are too often eaten when unripe. When ripe, they are as wholesome as any other fruit. Unripe they provoke choleraic diarrhoea.

The prune, a variety of dried plum, has been recommended as a remedy against viciousness and irritability. An American doctor declares that there is a certain medicinal property in the prune which acts directly upon the nervous system, and that is where the evil passions have their seat. He reports that he tried the experiment of including prunes in the meals of the vicious, intractable youths of a reformatory, and that by the end of a week they were peaceable as lambs. Most writers who comment on this seem to suggest that any fruit which is mildly aperient would produce the same effect. But the mother of a large family tells me that she has observed that prunes seem to possess a soothing property that is all their own.

Prune Tea.

Prune tea is an excellent drink for irritable persons. It is made as follows: To every pint of washed prunes allow 1 quart of distilled water. Soak the prunes all night, and afterwards simmer to rags in the same water. Strain, and flavour with lemon juice if desired.

Potato.

The potato is a cheap and homely remedy against gout, scurvy, and rickets. Dr. Lambe tells how he cured a case of scurvy solely with raw potatoes. One of the favourite dishes of that good old doctor was a salad composed of sliced raw potatoes and olive oil.

In order to preserve the medicinal properties of potatoes when cooked, they must always be steamed in their jackets. The skin may be removed before eating, but care should be taken not to allow a particle of the potato to adhere to it. The valuable potash salts chiefly lie just under the skin.

A raw potato scraped or powdered to a pulp is an excellent remedy for burns and scalds.

Dr. Fernie recommends the following decoction with which to bathe the swollen and inflamed joints of rheumatic sufferers. Take 1 lb. potatoes, cut each into four, but do not peel them. Boil in 2 pints of water until stewed down to 1 pint. Strain, and use the liquid.

Eaten to excess potatoes are apt to cause dullness and laziness.

Radish.

The radish is commonly cited as indigestible, but for all that it is commended by old writers as a potent remedy for stone. If not too old, well masticated, and eaten at the beginning of a meal, I do not think it is more indigestible than the majority of vegetables.

A syrup made with the juice expressed from pounded radishes and cane sugar is recommended for rheumatism, bronchial troubles, whooping-cough, and pustular eruptions.

Dr. Fernie notes that the black radish is especially useful against whooping-cough, probably by reason of its volatile, sulphureted oil. "It is employed in Germany for this purpose by cutting off the top, and then making a hole within the root, which hole is filled with treacle, or honey, and allowed to stand thus for two or three days; afterwards a teaspoonful of the medicated liquid is to be given two or three times in the day, with a dessertspoonful of water, when required."

I am not acquainted with the "black radish," but mothers might do worse, in cases of whooping-cough, than give their children the juice of pounded radishes mixed with pure honey.

Raspberry.

Raspberries are excellent against the scurvy, and, like the blackberry, good for relaxed bowels. They are a very wholesome fruit, and should be given to those who have "weak and queasy stomachs."

Rice.

The chief medicinal value of rice lies in the quickness with which it is digested. One authority says that "it can be taken four times a day and the patient still get twenty hours' rest." It is consequently of great value in digestive and intestinal troubles. But it should be unpolished, otherwise it is an ill-balanced, deficient food. It should likewise be boiled in only just enough soft water to be absorbed during the cooking. One cup of rice should be put on in a double saucepan with three cups of cold water and tightly covered. When the water is all absorbed the rice will be cooked.

The large-grained, unpolished rice sold at "Food-Reform" stores at 3d. per lb. absorbs the water and cooks much more easily than a smaller variety sold at 2d. I have found the latter most unsatisfactory.

Rhubarb.

Rhubarb is a wholesome and cooling spring vegetable, and may well take the place of cooked fruit when the latter is scarce. But it is generally forbidden to rheumatic and gouty patients on account of its oxalic acid. This oxalic acid is supposed to combine with the lime in the blood of the gouty person, and to form crystals of oxalate of lime, which are eliminated by the kidneys. At the same time the general health suffers. "Dr. Prout," writes Dr.

Fernie, "says he has seen well-marked instances in which an oxalate of lime kidney attack has followed the use of garden rhubarb in a tart or pudding, likewise of sorrel in a salad, particularly when at the same time the patient has been drinking hard water. But chemists explain that oxalates may be excreted in the urine without having necessarily been a constituent, as such, of vegetable or other foods taken at table, seeing that citric, malic, and other organic acids which are found distributed throughout the vegetable world are liable to chemical conversion into oxalic acid through a fermentation or perverted digestion."

I think the moral of the above is: "Do not drink hard water." Especially do not cook fruit and vegetables in hard water. They are nearly always rendered indigestible by such a process, and "vegetarianism," not the hard water, is often blamed for the sufferings of the consumers.

Rhubarb is apt to be over-valued as a "spring medicine" on account of its association with the Turkey rhubarb of materia medica. It should be thoroughly ripe before eating.

I am not recommending Turkey rhubarb.

Sage.

Sage is said to promote longevity, to quicken the senses and memory, and to strengthen the nerves.

Sage tea is recommended for pulmonary consumption and for excessive perspiration of the feet. A teaspoonful of dried sage, or rather more if the fresh leaves be used, is steeped in half a pint of water for twenty-four hours. A teacupful is to be taken night and morning.

Sage, like so many of the fragrant herbs, is antiseptic.

Strawberry.

The strawberry is exceptionally wholesome on account of its being so easily digested. It is recommended for gout, rheumatism, and the stone. Also for anemic patients on account of the iron it contains.

H. Benjafield, M.B., advises anemic girls to take 1 quart of strawberries per day, and when these are not obtainable several ripe bananas.

Spinach.

Professor Bunge declared that iron should never be taken in its mineral form, but that those who are in need of an iron tonic should take it as it exists in vegetables and fruit. To this end he especially commends spinach.

Dr. Luff puts spinach first on a list of vegetables recommended to those who suffer from gouty tendencies.

Spinach is very easily digested, and so juicy that no added water is needed in which to cook it.

Tomato.

The tomato, according to an American physician, is one of the most powerful deobstruents (remover of disease particles, and opener of the natural channels of the body) of the materia medica. It should be used in all affections of the liver, etc., where calomel is indicated.

The superstition that tomatoes are a cause of cancer is absolutely without foundation. Vegetarian cancer patients who have recovered after being given up as "hopeless" by the orthodox faculty eat tomatoes freely. Another belief, strongly supported by some otherwise "advanced" scientific men, is that tomatoes are bad for those who suffer from a tendency to gout, or uric acid disease. But this has been contradicted by others. The evil agency in the tomato is supposed to be the oxalic salt which it undoubtedly contains. But it has been shown by experiment how certain chemical compounds as obtained from plants act quite differently to the same compounds artificially prepared in the laboratory. So that the contention of those who assert that the tomato is not only harmless, but even beneficial to gouty subjects, is not unreasonable. Speaking from experience, I can only say that one of the goutiest subjects I know eats tomatoes nearly every day of his life, and continues to progress rapidly towards health.

A tomato poultice is said to cleanse foul ulcers, and promote their healing. It should be renewed frequently, and applied hot.

Turnip.

Turnips are anti-scorbutic.

An old remedy for chronic coughs was turnip juice boiled with sugar. The turnips were grated, the juice pressed out, and 2?ozs. candied sugar were allowed to 1 pint of juice. This was boiled until it slightly thickened. A teaspoonful to be taken several times a day.

The green turnip tops, steamed until tender, are a good "spring medicine."

Thyme.

The common garden thyme, used for flavouring, is credited with many virtues. It is said to inspire courage and enliven the spirits, and for this reason should be taken by melancholy persons. It is good against nervous headache, flatulence, and hysterical affections. It is antiseptic.

Walnuts.

The walnut has been called vegetable arsenic because of its curative value in eczema. An oil obtained from the kernel has been found of great service when applied externally in cases of skin diseases. The leaves of the walnut tree are also used for the same purpose, both externally and internally. One ounce of the leaves to 12 tablespoonfuls of boiling water make a tea, half a tea-cup of which may be taken several times a day. The affected parts should also be washed with it.

Walnuts, to be well masticated, have been given to gouty and rheumatic patients with great success. About one dozen per day is the quantity prescribed. It is possible that herein lies the secret of the fact that our ancestors invariably took walnuts with their wine.

The green, unripe walnut is useful for expelling worms.

Wheat.

Whole wheat is a perfect food. In the form of white flour, however, it is an imperfect, unbalanced food, on account of its deprivation of the valuable phosphates which exist in the bran. Rickets and malnutrition generally are the outcome of the habitual use of white flour, unless the loss of mineral matter is counter balanced by other foods.

Only the very finest wholemeal, such as "Artox," for example, should be used for making bread, etc. The ordinary coarse wholemeals are apt to produce intestinal irritation.

Cracked wheat, soaked overnight in water and boiled for a couple of hours, is a favourite prescription of American writers for habitual constipation. It may be obtained at most large "Food-Reform" stores.

Bran Tea.

Nervous or anemic persons will derive great benefit from a course of bran tea. It is made as follows:--To every cup of bran allow 2 cups distilled water. Well wash the bran in cold water; it is generally full of dust. Put in a saucepan with the cold distilled water, cover tightly, and boil for thirty minutes. Strain, and 41lavor with sugar and lemon juice to taste. Take a teacupful night and morning.

###

www.ingramcontent.com/pod-product-compliance
Lightning Source LLC
Chambersburg PA
CBHW072258200526
45168CB00016B/2141